ARTHRI-

Step By Step Exercises To Conquer Knee Arthritis, Revitalize Your Joints And Embrace Movements

BY JOHN P. MEYER

Table of Contents

INTRODUCTION

Once upon a time, there lived two individuals whose lives were profoundly affected by knee arthritis - Sarah and Noah. Both in their mid-50s, they had been friends since childhood, sharing countless adventures and memories. However, the onset of knee arthritis changed everything, casting a shadow over their active and vibrant lives.

For Sarah, an avid hiker and nature enthusiast, knee arthritis was a crushing blow. The sharp pain in her knees now limited her once exhilarating hikes through the lush mountains and serene valleys. The fear of aggravating her condition had replaced her passion for exploration. As the days passed, Sarah avoided her beloved trails, choosing instead to retreat to the comfort of her home, missing the beauty of nature that once brought her immense joy.

On the other hand, Noah, an enthusiastic runner and fitness enthusiast, found his world shrinking due to knee arthritis. The adrenaline rush he experienced during his daily runs had given way to aching knees and restricted movements. His dream of completing a marathon seemed like a distant memory as he struggled to cover even short distances. Noah's frustration mounted as he witnessed his stamina and endurance slipping away, and the helplessness consumed him.

One gloomy afternoon, Sarah and Noah happened to cross paths while strolling through the town square. Their faces mirrored the shared pain and the yearning for their active lives to return. Sensing their mutual struggles, they shared their stories on a nearby bench.

As Sarah poured out her heart about losing her beloved hikes, Noah empathized deeply, describing his battle with giving up his passion for running. In that moment of vulnerability, they realized they weren't alone in their fight against knee arthritis.

Their conversation soon turned to hope, as Sarah recalled reading about exercises designed explicitly for knee arthritis management. Intrigued, they decided to explore these exercises together, believing they could regain control of their lives.

They met the next day at the local community center, where a compassionate physical therapist, Emily, welcomed them warmly. Emily explained that knee arthritis management requires a holistic approach, encompassing exercises, lifestyle changes, and emotional support.

Under Emily's guidance, Sarah and Noah began their resilience journey, starting with gentle range of motion exercises. As they practiced ankle pumps, toe taps, quadriceps contractions, and hamstring stretches, they discovered the power of movement to alleviate pain and stiffness. Encouraged by each other's progress, they formed a bond built on mutual support and determination.

In the following weeks, Sarah and Noah embraced low-impact cardiovascular exercises, taking them to the pool for swimming and water aerobics. They explored the joys of cycling and elliptical training, cherishing every moment of physical activity their knees allowed. The support they provided each other became an unshakable pillar of strength, propelling them forward in their journey.

As they incorporated balancing and flexibility exercises into their routine, Sarah and Noah found a renewed sense of stability and mobility. They indulged in the beauty of yoga and tai chi, mastering single-leg stances and heel-to-toe walks. Their progress was slow but steady, and they celebrated each small victory with unwavering enthusiasm.

However, just like any journey, Sarah and Noah encountered challenges. Flare-ups and setbacks were inevitable, but they faced them with resilience and adaptability. They contacted their supportive network, seeking encouragement from friends, family, and their newfound support group for individuals with knee arthritis.

Tracking their progress and setting realistic long-term goals became a source of motivation for Sarah and Noah. They celebrated the milestones achieved, embracing non-scale victories as a testament to their unwavering commitment. Each step transformed their lives, and their outlook became more hopeful.

As the seasons changed, Sarah and Noah stood at the threshold of a life they had almost lost to knee arthritis. Their journey of overcoming challenges and staying motivated brought them closer as friends and as warriors of resilience.

One sunny afternoon, they found themselves at the starting line of a local charity walk. With tears of joy and gratitude, they clasped hands and embarked on the walk together. Crossing the finish line felt like crossing the threshold of a new beginning. Sarah and Noah realized that their journey of conquering knee arthritis had led them to a profound realization - that the human spirit, fueled by determination and supported by love, can overcome any obstacle.

And so, the tale of Sarah and Noah inspires all those facing knee arthritis. Their story reminds us that with the right exercises, a supportive network, and unwavering determination, we can conquer life's challenges. Let their resilience journey be a beacon of hope for all those striving to reclaim their lives and embrace the joy of movement once more.

In the end, the power of exercises for knee arthritis lies not only in healing the body but also in nurturing the spirit, allowing us to soar to new heights and savor life's precious moments.

CHAPTER ONE: UNDERSTANDING KNEE ARTHRITIS

Knee arthritis is a prevalent and often debilitating condition affecting millions of people worldwide. It involves the inflammation and degeneration of the knee joint, leading to pain, stiffness, and reduced mobility.

What Is Knee Arthritis?

Knee arthritis is a complex condition that affects the intricate structures of the knee joint, which connects the thigh bone (femur) to the shinbone (tibia). Walking, running, and bending are all necessary motions made possible by the knee joint, which functions as a pivotal hinge. Within the joint, a layer of cartilage acts as a cushion, reducing friction between the bones and ensuring smooth motion.

This protecting cartilage starts to deteriorate over time in knee arthritis, forcing the bones to scrape against one another. As a result, the knee joint becomes inflamed and painful, leading to stiffness and difficulty moving. While knee arthritis is commonly associated with aging, it can also occur due to injuries, genetic predisposition, and certain medical conditions.

Types Of Knee Arthritis

Understanding the different types of knee arthritis is essential for accurate diagnosis and tailored treatment plans. The most prevalent kinds of arthritis in the knee include:

1. **Osteoarthritis:** This is the most prevalent form of knee arthritis and is often associated with aging. As we age, the cartilage naturally deteriorates, leading to osteoarthritis. Although it can happen to younger people as well, it most frequently affects those over the age of 50, especially if there is a history of joint injuries or other risk factors.

2. **Rheumatoid Arthritis:** This, in contrast to osteoarthritis, is an inflammatory condition. Inflammation and cartilage damage result when the immune system mistakenly targets the synovium, the lining of the joint. Rheumatoid arthritis can affect multiple joints in the body, including the knees, and is more commonly observed in women.

3. **Post-Traumatic Arthritis:** After a severe knee injury, such as a fracture, ligament rupture, or meniscus injury, this kind of arthritis develops. The initial trauma to the knee joint can lead to long-term joint damage, eventually resulting in post-traumatic arthritis.

Causes and Risk Factors

Various factors influence the development of knee arthritis, and understanding these causes and risk factors is essential for prevention and effective management. The following are some of the main causes and risk factors for knee arthritis:

1. **Age:** As mentioned earlier, aging raises the likelihood of developing knee arthritis, mostly because of the typical tear and damage that develops over time.

2. **Genetics:** Family history can play a role in the development of knee arthritis. If you have a family member with knee arthritis, you may also be at a higher risk of developing the condition.

3. **Weight:** Excess body weight puts additional stress on the knees, increasing the risk of knee arthritis. The stress on the knee joints can be lessened by maintaining a healthy weight.

4. **Joint Injuries:** Previous knee injuries, such as fractures or ligament tears, can lead to post-traumatic arthritis, as they may cause long-term joint damage.

5. **Repetitive Stress:** Jobs or activities that require lengthy standing or frequent kneeling can contribute to the development of knee arthritis over time.

6. **Infections or Diseases:** Infections or underlying conditions like gout can also contribute to the development of knee arthritis.

Signs And Symptoms

Recognizing the signs and symptoms of knee arthritis is crucial for early diagnosis and intervention. Common symptoms of knee arthritis include:

1. **Joint Pain:** Pain in the knee joint, often described as a dull ache, can significantly indicate knee arthritis. The pain may worsen with movement or prolonged activity.

2. **Stiffness:** Individuals with knee arthritis may experience stiffness in the knee joint, particularly after periods of inactivity or upon waking up in the morning.

3. **Swelling:** Inflammation in the knee joint can cause swelling and tenderness, making it sensitive to touch.

4. **Reduced Range of Motion:** As knee arthritis progresses, individuals may notice a decrease in the knee joint's range of motion, making it challenging to bend or straighten the knee fully.

5. **Crepitus:** Some people may experience a grating or grinding sensation in the knee joint when moving, known as crepitus.

6. **Instability:** A feeling of the knee giving way or being unstable during weight-bearing activities.

7. **Warmth and Redness:** The knee may feel warm to the touch and appear red due to inflammation.

It's essential to note that symptoms can vary from person to person and may worsen over time if left untreated.

Diagnosing Knee Arthritis

Diagnosing knee arthritis involves a comprehensive evaluation by a healthcare professional. The following steps are often part of the diagnostic process:

1. **Medical History:** The healthcare provider will inquire about the individual's medical history, including any previous knee injuries, family history of arthritis, and the nature of the symptoms.

2. **Physical Examination:** A medical evaluation of the knee joint will be conducted to assess the range of motion, stability, and signs of inflammation.

3. **Imaging Tests:** X-rays, MRI scans, and ultrasound may be used to obtain detailed images of the knee joint. These imaging tests can reveal cartilage damage, bone changes, and other signs of knee arthritis.

4. **Joint Fluid Analysis:** In some cases, a procedure known as joint fluid analysis (arthrocentesis) may be performed to examine the synovial fluid in the knee joint. This analysis can help rule out other conditions and determine if there is inflammation present.

Conclusion: Understanding knee arthritis is crucial for individuals affected by this condition and their caregivers. By exploring its causes, types, symptoms, and diagnostic process, we can empower readers to take proactive steps in managing knee arthritis effectively.

Early detection and appropriate exercises and treatments can improve joint function and overall quality of life for those with knee arthritis. This book has aimed to provide a comprehensive overview of knee arthritis, emphasizing the importance of exercise and proper care in managing this prevalent joint disorder.

CHAPTER TWO: THE IMPORTANCE OF EXERCISE IN MANAGING KNEE ARTHRITIS

Knee arthritis can be a life-altering condition, causing pain, stiffness, and reduced mobility. However, there is a silver lining: exercise can be pivotal in managing knee arthritis and improving overall joint health. This chapter aims to delve into the importance of exercise as a cornerstone of knee arthritis management, exploring how exercise helps, its myriad benefits, and dispelling common misconceptions that may deter individuals from engaging in physical activity.

How Exercise Helps In Knee Arthritis Management

The notion of exercise might seem daunting for those living with knee arthritis, as pain and stiffness can make physical activity appear challenging. However, understanding the importance of exercise is crucial for individuals seeking relief from knee arthritis symptoms. Exercise can help maintain joint function, strengthen surrounding muscles, and improve overall well-being.

Regular physical activity can prevent muscle weakening and joint stiffness, empowering individuals to retain their independence and enjoy a higher quality of life. By understanding the significance of exercise in knee arthritis management, individuals can embrace movement as an essential component of their treatment plan.

It's vital to comprehend how exercise positively impacts knee arthritis management. Engaging in appropriate activities can offer a multitude of benefits, such as:

1. **Strengthening Muscles:** Specific exercises target the muscles surrounding the knee joint, enhancing joint stability and reducing the strain on the affected area.

2. **Improving Joint Flexibility:** Gentle exercises can increase the knee's range of motion, allowing for more comfortable and fluid movements.

3. **Weight Management:** Regular physical activity aids in weight management, alleviating the stress placed on the knee joint and slowing down cartilage degeneration.

4. **Enhancing Joint Lubrication:** Synovial fluid, a natural lubricant that facilitates joint movement and lowers friction, is stimulated by movement.

5. **Mood Enhancement:** Exercise releases endorphins, which improves mood and aids in coping with the

psychological effects of chronic illnesses like knee arthritis.

Understanding how exercise contributes to knee arthritis management enables people to decide for themselves what kind of physical activity is best for them, leading to improved joint health and overall wellness.

Benefits Of Exercise For Knee Arthritis

The benefits of exercise for knee arthritis are far-reaching, encompassing physical and emotional aspects. Some of the notable advantages include:

1. **Pain Relief:** Doing appropriate exercises can reduce knee pain and discomfort, making daily activities more manageable.
2. **Increased Mobility:** Regular movement helps improve joint flexibility and range of motion, enabling individuals to perform everyday tasks more efficiently.
3. **Enhanced Muscle Strength:** Strengthening exercises target the muscles supporting the knee joint, leading to improved joint stability and decreased stress on the knee.

4. **Weight Control:** Exercise aids in weight management, preventing excessive pressure on the knee joint and slowing the progression of arthritis.

5. **Improved Sleep:** Regular physical activity can promote better sleep patterns, improving overall health and well-being.

6. **Reduced Depression and Anxiety:** The endorphins released during exercise act as natural mood enhancers, reducing symptoms of depression and anxiety commonly associated with chronic conditions.

7. **Better Overall Health:** Exercise positively affects cardiovascular health, bone density, and immune function, contributing to a healthier lifestyle.

By embracing exercise and recognizing its multifaceted benefits, individuals can take an active role in managing knee arthritis and regaining control of their lives.

Addressing Common Misconceptions About Exercise And Arthritis

Despite the numerous benefits of exercise for knee arthritis, several misconceptions may discourage individuals from engaging in physical activity. Addressing and dispelling these misconceptions is essential for promoting a positive and informed approach to exercise:

- **Misconception:** Exercise worsens arthritis pain.
  Fact: When done correctly and under appropriate guidance, exercise can alleviate knee arthritis pain and improve joint function.
- **Misconception:** Individuals with knee arthritis should avoid physical activity altogether.
  Fact: Carefully chosen in consultation with a healthcare professional, low-impact exercises are safe and beneficial for knee arthritis management.
- **Misconception:** Exercise leads to joint damage.
  Fact: Properly prescribed exercises help strengthen muscles, aid the knee joint and lower the chance of joint injury.
- **Misconception:** Rest is the best remedy for knee arthritis.
  Fact: While rest is essential, excessive inactivity can lead to muscle weakening and joint stiffness, exacerbating knee arthritis symptoms.
- **Misconception:** Only high-intensity workouts are effective.

Fact: Gentle, low-impact exercises can be highly effective in managing knee arthritis and improving joint health.

Conclusion: Exercise is fundamental to knee arthritis management, offering many physical and emotional benefits. By embracing movement and understanding its positive impact, individuals with knee arthritis can lead more fulfilling lives filled with reduced pain, increased mobility, and enhanced overall well-being.

By dispelling common misconceptions, we aim to empower individuals to take an active role in their knee arthritis management, ensuring that exercise becomes an integral part of their journey toward improved joint health and a more fulfilling life.

Remember, with the right exercises, guidance, and dedication; movement is often a strong ally in the fight against knee arthritis.

CHAPTER THREE: PREPARING FOR YOUR EXERCISE JOURNEY

Embarking on an exercise journey to manage knee arthritis is an empowering step towards improved joint health and overall well-being. However, proper preparation and guidance are essential for a safe and practical experience before diving into physical activity.

Before starting your exercise program, this chapter will explore crucial steps, including consulting your healthcare professional, assessing your current condition, setting realistic exercise goals, and considering safety precautions to ensure a successful and fulfilling exercise journey.

Consulting Your Healthcare Professional

Before beginning any exercise regimen, it is vital to consult your healthcare professional, such as your primary care physician or a rheumatologist, especially if you have knee arthritis. These professionals possess the expertise to assess your medical history, current condition, and potential risk factors, enabling them to provide personalized recommendations for exercise.

Your healthcare provider will evaluate the severity of your knee arthritis, any existing joint damage, and any related health conditions that might influence your exercise choices. This assessment will help determine the exercises most suitable for your individual needs, ensuring that your exercise journey aligns with your overall health goals.

Additionally, your healthcare professional can offer valuable insights into exercises that will strengthen the muscles around your knee joint, enhance joint stability, and improve your range of motion while minimizing the risk of exacerbating your knee arthritis symptoms.

Assessing Your Current Condition

Understanding your current physical condition is crucial before starting any exercise program. Conducting a self-assessment allows you to gauge your abilities, limitations, and potential areas of improvement. Begin by observing your knee arthritis symptoms, noting the intensity of pain, stiffness, and swelling experienced regularly.

Assess your joint flexibility and range of motion, paying attention to any specific movements that cause discomfort or difficulty. Identifying your physical strengths and limitations will guide you in selecting exercises that align with your abilities while addressing areas that require improvement.

To further assess your current condition, consider engaging in a few simple exercises recommended by your healthcare professional. Take note of how your body responds to each movement, and do not hesitate to communicate any discomfort or concerns to your healthcare provider.

Creating Realistic Exercise Goals

Setting realistic exercise goals is a crucial aspect of your exercise journey. While the desire to achieve immediate results might be substantial, it is essential to approach exercise with patience and long-term objectives. Realistic goals can help prevent frustration and injury while promoting steady progress and success.

When creating exercise goals, consider both short-term and long-term objectives. Short-term goals can be daily or weekly targets focusing on consistency and adherence to your exercise routine. For example, aiming to complete a set of specific exercises three times a week might be a manageable short-term goal.

Long-term goals, however, could span several months and involve improvements in joint flexibility, increased strength, or enhanced endurance. Be sure to communicate these goals with your healthcare professional, as they can provide guidance and support throughout your exercise journey.

Remember that each individual's journey is unique, and progress may vary from person to person. Celebrate your achievements, no matter how small, as they contribute to your overall well-being and journey towards better knee arthritis management.

Safety Considerations And Precautions

Safety is paramount when engaging in any exercise routine, especially for individuals with knee arthritis. Taking necessary precautions can prevent injuries, manage pain, and ensure a positive exercise experience.

- **Warm-up and Cool-down:** Always begin your exercise session with a gentle warm-up to prepare your muscles and joints for physical activity. Simple movements like leg swings, gentle stretches, or a short walk can help increase muscle blood flow and reduce the risk of injury. Similarly, conclude your exercise routine with a cool-down to gradually reduce your heart rate and prevent muscle stiffness.

- **Appropriate Footwear:** Proper footwear with adequate support is essential for individuals with knee arthritis. Shoes that offer cushioning and stability can help absorb impact during exercise, reducing stress on the knee joint. Consult a podiatrist or knowledgeable shoe salesperson to find the best footwear for your exercise needs.

- **Low-Impact Exercises:** For individuals with knee arthritis, low-impact exercises are generally safer and more manageable. Activities like swimming, cycling, and elliptical training place less stress on the knee joint while providing excellent cardiovascular benefits. Gradually incorporate higher-impact exercises, such as jogging or jumping, once you have built sufficient strength and flexibility.

- **Avoid Overexertion:** Listen to your body during exercise, and do not push yourself beyond your limits. Overexertion can strain the knee joint and lead to increased pain and inflammation. Gradually progress your exercise routine, allowing your body ample time to adapt and grow stronger.

- **Rest and Recovery:** These are essential for muscle repair and joint health. Be mindful of how your body responds to exercise, and schedule rest days to prevent overuse injuries. Consult your healthcare professional for guidance if you experience persistent pain or swelling after exercise.

Conclusion: Preparing for your exercise journey is crucial to effectively managing knee arthritis and improving joint health. By consulting your healthcare professional, assessing your current condition, setting realistic exercise goals, and considering safety precautions, you can embark on a safe and fulfilling exercise routine tailored to your individual needs.

Remember, patience and dedication are crucial to progressing in your exercise journey. Stay consistent, celebrate your achievements, and embrace the positive changes that regular exercise can bring. By nurturing your body through exercise, you are taking proactive steps towards better knee arthritis management and a more vibrant and active lifestyle.

CHAPTER FOUR: GENTLE RANGE OF MOTION EXERCISES

In the journey to managing knee arthritis effectively, gentle range of motion exercises plays a pivotal role in maintaining joint flexibility, reducing stiffness, and improving overall knee function.

These exercises are designed to be low-impact and safe, making them ideal for individuals with knee arthritis seeking to enhance their joint health without exacerbating their symptoms.

This chapter will explore five essential gentle range of motion exercises for knee arthritis: ankle pumps and toe taps, quadriceps contractions, hamstring stretches, calf raises, leg raises, and knee extensions.

Ankle Pumps And Toe Taps

Ankle pumps and toe taps are simple yet effective range-of-motion exercises that target the ankles and toes, promoting joint mobility and circulation. These exercises are particularly beneficial for individuals with knee arthritis, as they can be performed while seated or lying down, reducing knee stress.

Instructions

1. Ankle Pumps:

a. Sit or lie down with your legs extended.

b. Slowly flex your ankles, pointing your toes towards your body.

c. Hold the bent position for a few seconds. d. Slowly return to the starting position. e. Now, slowly extend your ankles, pointing your toes away from your body. f. Hold the extended position for a few seconds. g. Repeat the ankle pumps for 10-15 repetitions.

2. Toe Taps:

a. Sit or lie down with your legs extended.

b. Lift your toes off the ground, keeping your heels in contact with the surface.

c. Lower your toes back down.

d. Raise your heels off the floor at this time, keeping your toes in touch with the surface.

e. Lower your heels back down.

f. Repeat the toe taps for 10-15 repetitions.

Regularly performing ankle pumps and toe taps can help improve ankle flexibility, increase blood flow to the lower extremities, and enhance the overall joint range of motion.

Quadriceps Contractions

Strengthening the quadriceps muscles at the front of the thighs is vital for knee arthritis management. Strong quadriceps help support the knee joint and reduce strain during weight-bearing activities. Quadriceps contractions are gentle isometric exercises performed while seated or lying down.

Instructions

1. **Seated Quadriceps Contractions:**
   a. Sit on a chair with your feet flat on the ground.
   b. Tighten the muscles at the front of your thigh (quadriceps) lowering your knee into the chair.
   c. Hold the contraction for 5-10 seconds.
   d. Release and relax the muscles.
   e. Repeat the seated quadriceps contractions for 10-15 repetitions.

2. **Supine Quadriceps Contractions:**
   a. Lie down on your back with your legs extended.
   b. Tighten the quadriceps muscles in your affected leg by pushing the back of your knee down into the floor or mat.
   c. Hold the contraction for 5-10 seconds.
   d. Release and relax the muscles.

e. Repeat the supine quadriceps contractions for 10-15 repetitions on each leg.

Incorporating regular quadriceps contractions into your exercise routine can help improve knee stability, reduce knee pain, and enhance functional strength for daily activities.

Hamstring Stretches

Hamstring stretches are essential for maintaining balanced muscle strength around the knee joint, particularly in individuals with knee arthritis. These stretches focus on the muscles at the back of the thighs, promoting flexibility and reducing tension in the hamstring muscles.

Instructions

1. **Standing Hamstring Stretch:**
a. Stand upright with your feet hip-width apart.
b. Step your affected leg back slightly, keeping both feet pointing forward.
c. Bend your front knee slightly and hinge at the hips, reaching your hands towards your front foot.
d. Feel the stretch along the back of your extended leg (hamstring).

e.   Hold the stretch for 20-30 seconds while maintaining a gentle bend in the front knee.

f.   Return to the starting position.

g.   Repeat the standing hamstring stretch on each leg for 2-3 repetitions.

2.   **Seated Hamstring Stretch:**

a.   Your feet should be flat on the floor as you sit on the edge of a chair.

b.   Extend your affected leg in front of you, keeping your heel on the floor.

c.   Lean forward slightly from your hips, reaching towards your toes with your hands.

d.   Feel the stretch along the back of your extended leg.

e.   Hold the stretch for 20-30 seconds.

f.   Return to the starting position.

g.   Repeat the seated hamstring stretch on each leg for 2-3 repetitions.

Including hamstring stretches in your exercise routine can improve hamstring flexibility, reduce muscle tension, and enhance knee joint mobility.

Calf Raises

Calf raises are gentle exercises that target the calf muscles, providing support for the ankles and knees. Strengthening the calves can help improve overall lower limb stability and balance, which is crucial for individuals with knee arthritis seeking to engage in weight-bearing activities.

Instructions

1. **Standing Calf Raises:**
   a. Stand upright with your feet hip-width apart and your hands resting on a stable surface, such as a chair or wall, for support.
   b. Pushing your heels off the ground, steadily elevate onto the balls of your feet.
   c. Hold the raised position for 2-3 seconds.
   d. Gently lower your heels back down to the ground.
   e. Repeat the standing calf raises for 10-15 repetitions.
2. **Seated Calf Raises:**
   a. Sit on a chair with your feet flat on the ground.
   b. Lift your heels off the ground, rising up onto the balls of your feet.
   c. Hold the raised position for 2-3 seconds.
   d. Lower your heels back down to the ground.

e. Repeat the seated calf raises for 10-15 repetitions.

Regularly performing calf raises can contribute to increased muscle strength, better ankle stability, and reduced knee strain during weight-bearing activities.

Leg Raises And Knee Extensions

Leg raises, and knee extensions are gentle exercises that target the quadriceps muscles while promoting knee joint stability and flexibility. These exercises are suitable for individuals with knee arthritis, as they can be performed while lying down, eliminating pressure on the knees.

Instructions

1. **Straight Leg Raise:**
   a. One leg should be extended, and the other should be bent at the knee as you lay on your back.
   b. Slowly lift your extended leg off the ground, keeping it straight.
   c. Hold the raised position for 2-3 seconds.
   d. Gently lower your leg back down to the ground.
   e. Repeat the straight leg raise for 10-15 repetitions on each leg.

2. Knee Extension:

a. Sit on a chair with your feet flat on the ground.

b. Extend your affected leg out straight in front of you.

c. Lift your foot off the ground, straightening your knee as much as possible.

d. Hold the extended position for 2-3 seconds.

e. Gently lower your foot back down to the ground.

f. Repeat the knee extension for 10-15 repetitions on each leg.

Leg raises and knee extensions are valuable exercises for strengthening the quadriceps muscles, enhancing knee stability, and improving overall lower limb function.

Conclusion: Gentle range of motion exercises are invaluable tools for individuals with knee arthritis seeking to manage their condition and improve joint health. Ankle pumps and toe taps, quadriceps contractions, hamstring stretches, calf raises, leg raises, and knee extensions are essential components of an exercise routine designed to maintain joint flexibility, strengthen supporting muscles, and enhance overall knee function.

These low-impact exercises are safe and effective, allowing individuals to experience the benefits of regular physical activity without placing excessive strain on the knees. As with any exercise program, it is crucial to consult your healthcare professional before starting these exercises to ensure they suit your specific condition and overall health.

Incorporating a gentle range of motion exercises into your daily routine can contribute to better knee arthritis management, reduced pain, and increased mobility. Stay committed to your exercise journey, and remember that progress may be gradual but rewarding. Embrace movement, prioritize self-care, and savor the positive changes these gentle exercises can bring.

CHAPTER FIVE: STRENGTHENING EXERCISES FOR KNEE STABILITY

Strengthening the muscles surrounding the knee joint is fundamental to managing knee arthritis and improving joint stability. Engaging in targeted strengthening exercises can alleviate knee pain and enhance overall joint function and support. This chapter will explore five essential strengthening exercises for knee stability: wall slides, step-ups and step-downs, resistance band exercises, leg presses, bridges and hip abductions

Wall Slides

Wall slides are an effective strengthening exercise that targets the quadriceps muscles, which play a crucial role in knee stability. This workout strengthens and lengthens the quadriceps, supporting the knee joint during weight-bearing activities.

Instructions

1. Your feet should be shoulder-width apart as you stand with your back pressed against a wall.

2. Kneel on the wall and descend it, ensuring your knees are aligned with your ankles and not going past your toes.

3. If you cannot go that low, lower yourself until your thighs are parallel to the ground or at a comfortable level.

4. Hold the position for 5-10 seconds, then push through your heels to return to the starting position.

5. Repeat the wall slides for 10-15 repetitions.

To maximize the exercise's benefits and reduce the danger of injury, it is crucial to maintain appropriate form and control throughout.

Step-ups And Step-downs

Step-ups and step-downs are functional exercises that target the quadriceps, hamstrings, and gluteal muscles, enhancing overall lower limb strength and knee stability. Performing these exercises can improve balance and coordination, making them beneficial for daily activities that involve stair climbing or walking on uneven surfaces.

Instructions

1. **Step-ups:**

a. Stand in front of a sturdy step or elevated surface.

b. Step onto the surface with your affected leg, ensuring your entire foot is securely on the step.

c. Push through your heel and lift your body up onto the step.

d. Hold the position for a few seconds, then step back down with the same leg.

e. Repeat the step-ups for 10-15 repetitions on each leg.

2. Step-downs:

a. Stand on the elevated surface with your affected leg.

b. Lower your body down gently, ensuring your entire foot is on the surface.

c. Control the movement and use your muscles to lower your body with stability.

d. Step back up with the same leg and repeat the step-downs for 10-15 repetitions on each leg.

Performing step-ups and step-downs can help build strength and stability in the lower extremities, reducing the risk of knee injuries during daily activities.

Resistance Band Exercises

The tendons and muscles supporting the knee joint can be strengthened with resistance band workouts, which are adaptable and efficient. These exercises provide progressive resistance, allowing individuals to customize the intensity of their workout based on their current abilities.

Instructions

1. **Seated Leg Extensions with Resistance Band:**
   a. Sit on a chair with your feet flat on the ground and a resistance band tied around your ankles.
   b. Extend your affected leg forward against the resistance of the band.
   c. Hold the extended position for a few seconds before slowly returning to the starting position.
   d. Repeat the seated leg extensions for 10-15 repetitions on each leg.

2. **Clamshells with Resistance Band:**
   a. Place a resistance band fastened around your legs right above the knees as you lay on one side with your knees bent.
   b. Keeping your feet together, open your knees like a clamshell while maintaining tension on the band.
   c. Hold the open position for a few seconds before slowly closing your knees.
   d. Repeat the clamshells for 10-15 repetitions on each side.

Resistance band exercises can target various muscle groups around the knee joint, enhancing stability and functional strength.

Leg Presses

Leg presses are gym-based exercises that specifically target the quadriceps, hamstrings, and gluteal muscles. This exercise requires a leg press machine commonly found in fitness centers, making it a valuable addition to a comprehensive knee arthritis management program.

Instructions

1. Put your feet flat on the footplate of the leg press machine as you sit down and your knees bent 90 degrees.
2. Legs should be straightened without locking, and you should push the footplate farther from your body.
3. Hold the extended position for a few seconds, then in order to get back to the beginning position, softly bend your knees.
4. Repeat the leg presses for 10-15 repetitions.

Adjusting the leg press machine to a comfortable starting position is essential for maximizing the effectiveness of this exercise and minimizing strain on the knee joint.

Bridges And Hip Abductions

Bridges and hip abductions are excellent exercises for strengthening the gluteal muscles and stabilizing the hips, which is essential for overall lower limb function and knee stability.

Instructions

1. **Bridges:**
   a. Your feet should be flat on the ground as you lay on your back with your knees bent.
   b. Establish an even line from your shoulders to your knees by pressing through your heels and lifting your hips off the ground.
   c. Hold the bridge position for a few seconds before lowering your hips back down to the ground.
   d. Repeat the bridges for 10-15 repetitions.

2. **Hip Abductions:**
   a. Lie on your side with your legs stacked on top of each other.

b. Lift your top leg away from your body, leading with your heel, while keeping your hips stacked.

c. Hold the lifted position for a few seconds before lowering your leg back down.

d. Repeat the hip abductions for 10-15 repetitions on each side.

Bridges and hip abductions can help improve hip stability, reduce the risk of knee pain, and enhance overall lower limb strength.

Conclusion: Incorporating strengthening exercises for knee stability into your exercise routine can significantly improve knee arthritis management and overall joint function.

Wall slides, step-ups and step-downs, resistance band exercises, leg presses, bridges, and hip abductions are valuable additions to a well-rounded exercise program, concentrating on the main muscle groups that protect and support the knee joint.

When performing these exercises, it is crucial to prioritize proper form and technique to prevent injuries and ensure optimal benefits. Remember to consult your healthcare professional before beginning any new exercise regimen, especially if you have knee arthritis, to receive personalized guidance and recommendations.

Consistency and dedication to your strengthening exercises will improve knee stability, reduce pain, and enhance overall mobility. Embrace the power of exercise in your knee arthritis management journey, and witness its positive impact on your quality of life.

CHAPTER SIX: LOW-IMPACT CARDIOVASCULAR EXERCISES

Maintaining cardiovascular health is vital for individuals with knee arthritis, but high-impact activities can be challenging and potentially harmful to the knees. Low-impact cardiovascular exercises provide an excellent alternative, allowing individuals to elevate their heart rate, improve circulation, and enhance cardiovascular endurance without subjecting the knee joints to excessive stress.

This chapter will explore five low-impact cardiovascular exercises suitable for individuals with knee arthritis: swimming and water aerobics, cycling and stationary biking, elliptical training, rowing, and modified jogging and walking.

Swimming And Water Aerobics

Swimming and water aerobics are among the most effective low-impact cardiovascular exercises, offering many benefits for individuals with knee arthritis. The buoyancy of water reduces the impact on the joints, making these activities gentle on the knees while providing a full-body workout.

Instructions:

1. Swimming:

a. Choose your preferred swimming stroke (freestyle, breaststroke, backstroke, or butterfly).

b. As you warm up, start out softly and gradually pick up the speed.

c. Focus on maintaining proper form and breathing rhythm throughout your swim.

d. Aim for at least 20-30 minutes of continuous swimming to elevate your heart rate and improve cardiovascular endurance.

2. Water Aerobics:

a. Join a water aerobics class or perform water aerobics exercises in a shallow pool.

b. Engage in movements such as leg kicks, arm circles, jumping jacks, and squats, all while being supported by the water.

c. For a beneficial cardiovascular workout, perform the water aerobics routine for 30-45 minutes.

Swimming and water aerobics are gentle on the knees, making them excellent choices for individuals seeking to improve their cardiovascular fitness without causing discomfort or exacerbating knee arthritis symptoms.

Cycling And Stationary Biking

Cycling and stationary biking are low-impact cardiovascular exercises that effectively elevate the heart rate and strengthen the lower body muscles. Stationary biking, in particular, allows individuals to control the intensity of their workout while minimizing joint impact.

Instructions:

1. **Cycling:**
   a. If cycling outdoors, choose flat terrain or gentle inclines to reduce knee stress.
   b. Start with a warm-up, pedaling comfortably for 5-10 minutes.
   c. Gradually increase your speed and resistance to elevate your heart rate.
   d. Aim for 30-45 minutes of continuous cycling, alternating between faster and slower segments to challenge yourself.
2. **Stationary Biking:**
   a. Adjust the seat height and handlebar position for proper alignment and comfort.
   b. Begin with a warm-up by pedaling steadily for 5-10 minutes.

c. Increase the resistance on the stationary bike to intensify your workout.

d. Cycle for 30-45 minutes, varying your speed and resistance throughout the session.

Cycling and stationary biking are excellent low-impact exercises that provide cardiovascular benefits and help improve lower limb strength without putting excessive strain on the knee joints.

Elliptical Training

Popular low-impact cardiovascular workout known as elliptical training imitates the motion of walking or jogging without putting undue strain on the joints. This exercise targets the lower body muscles while providing an effective cardiovascular workout.

Instructions:

1. Stand on the elliptical machine with your feet flat on the foot pedals.
2. Hold the handles or use the handrails for balance.
3. Begin pedaling forward in a smooth and controlled motion.

4. Gradually increase your pace and resistance to elevate your heart rate.

5. Aim for 30-45 minutes of continuous elliptical training, focusing on proper form and maintaining a consistent pace.

Elliptical training is a joint-friendly option for individuals with knee arthritis, allowing them to engage in a challenging cardiovascular workout without the risk of impact-related discomfort.

Rowing

Rowing is a full-body, low-impact cardiovascular exercise that engages upper and lower body muscles. This exercise provides an excellent way to improve cardiovascular endurance and strengthen the core, arms, and legs.

Instructions:

1. Sit on the rowing machine with your feet securely placed on the footrests and your knees slightly bent.

2. Hold the rowing handle with an overhand grip, keeping your wrists straight.

3. Pull the rowing grip towards your torso while stretching your legs and pushing through your heels.

4. Bring the handle towards your body by leaning back slightly and contracting your abs.

5. Reverse the movement, bending your knees and leaning forward to return to the starting position.

6. Continue rowing for 30-45 minutes, maintaining a steady and controlled pace.

For people with knee arthritis who want to increase their level of fitness and general joint health, rowing is a great low-impact cardiovascular workout choice.

Modified Jogging And Walking

Jogging and walking can be modified to become low-impact cardiovascular exercises, allowing individuals with knee arthritis to enjoy the benefits of these activities without placing excessive strain on the knees.

Instructions:

1. **Modified Jogging:**

a. Find a soft surface, such as a grassy area or a track with a rubberized surface, to reduce impact.

b. Begin with a gentle warm-up, walking briskly for 5-10 minutes.

c. Transition into a slow jog, lifting your feet slightly off the ground with each step.

d. Keep the stride short and controlled to minimize the impact on the knees.

e. Jog for 10-15 minutes, gradually increasing the duration as your endurance improves.

f. Finish with a cool-down, walking slowly for 5-10 minutes.

2. **Walking:**

a. Choose supportive and cushioned footwear to absorb impact and reduce knee strain.

b. Start with a warm-up, walking moderately for 5-10 minutes.

c. Maintain a steady walking pace, swinging your arms for added momentum.

d. Aim for at least 30-45 minutes of continuous walking for a beneficial cardiovascular workout.

e. Incorporate walking into your daily routine, aiming for 10,000 steps per day to enhance overall cardiovascular health.

Modified jogging and walking are excellent low-impact cardiovascular exercises, allowing individuals to improve their fitness level and cardiovascular endurance at a comfortable and manageable pace for their knees.

Conclusion: Low-impact cardiovascular exercises provide an excellent means of improving cardiovascular health and overall fitness for individuals with knee arthritis. Swimming and water aerobics, cycling and stationary biking, elliptical training, rowing, and modified jogging and walking are all joint-friendly options that offer cardiovascular benefits without causing excessive knee stress.

Incorporating these low-impact exercises into your regular exercise routine can enhance cardiovascular endurance, strengthen supporting muscles, and improve joint function. As always, consult your healthcare professional before beginning any new exercise program, especially if you have knee arthritis, to ensure that these activities are safe and appropriate for your needs.

By prioritizing cardiovascular health through low-impact exercises, individuals with knee arthritis can enjoy the rewards of improved fitness, reduced pain, and a more active and vibrant lifestyle.

CHAPTER SEVEN: BALANCING AND FLEXIBILITY EXERCISES

Balancing and flexibility exercises are crucial in managing knee arthritis, promoting joint stability, and enhancing overall mobility. These exercises focus on improving balance, coordination, and flexibility, essential for reducing the risk of falls and maintaining optimal joint function.

This chapter will explore five critical balancing and flexibility exercises for knee arthritis: yoga and Tai Chi, single-leg stance and balance exercises, heel-to-toe walks, quadriceps stretch, and IT band stretch.

Yoga And Tai Chi For Knee Arthritis

These are ancient practices that offer numerous benefits for individuals with knee arthritis. These mind-body exercises combine controlled movements, deep breathing, and mindfulness to promote balance, flexibility, and well-being.

Yoga for Knee Arthritis

Yoga is a gentle yet effective practice that helps improve joint flexibility and strength. It focuses on various poses and stretches that target specific muscle groups, including those around the knee joint. Yoga can also aid in stress reduction and relaxation, which can be helpful in controlling knee arthritis pain.

Instructions:

- Begin with simple yoga poses that do not strain the knees excessively, such as Child's Pose, Cat-Cow Pose, and Seated Forward Bend.
- Progress to standing poses like Warrior II, Triangle Pose, and Tree Pose, which can help strengthen the legs and improve balance.
- Avoid deep knee bends or poses that cause knee discomfort or pain.
- Practice yoga regularly to experience its cumulative benefits for knee arthritis management.

Tai Chi for Knee Arthritis

Tai Chi is a slow and flowing martial art that promotes balance, flexibility, and inner calm. The gentle and controlled movements are particularly beneficial for individuals with knee arthritis, as they do not involve high-impact actions.

Instructions:

- Learn a Tai Chi routine from a certified instructor, focusing on the foundational movements and postures.
- Perform the routine slowly and mindfully, paying attention to your body's alignment and breathing.
- The controlled movements in Tai Chi can help improve knee stability and balance while reducing stress and tension.

Single-Leg Stance And Balance Exercises

Single-leg stance and balance exercises are designed to improve stability and proprioception, which is the body's ability to sense its position in space. These exercises are essential for reducing falls and enhancing knee-supporting muscle strength.

Instructions:

1. **Single-Leg Stance:**
- Stand next to a sturdy surface, such as a countertop or chair, for support.

- Using the other leg as support, raise one foot off the ground.
- Hold the single-leg stance for 10-20 seconds, gradually increasing the duration as you gain confidence and stability.
- Repeat on the other leg.
- Perform 10-15 repetitions on each leg.

2. **Balancing Exercises:**

- Stand with your feet shoulder-width apart.
- Put all of your weight on one leg, then raise the other one.
- Hold the lifted position for a few seconds, maintaining your balance.
- Get back to the beginning position and repeat with the opposite leg.
- Practice different balancing exercises, such as leg swings, leg circles, and standing hip abduction, to challenge your balance and stability.

Regularly practicing single-leg stance and balancing exercises can help improve proprioception, enhance knee stability, and lower the chance of falls in those with knee arthritis.

Heel-To-Toe Walks

Heel-to-toe walks, also known as tandem walks, are excellent exercises for improving balance and coordination. They challenge the body's stability and encourage controlled movement.

Instructions:

- Find a straight and clear path to walk along.
- Place one foot directly in front of the other, with the heel of the forward foot touching the toes of the back foot.
- Take slow and deliberate steps, maintaining the heel-to-toe alignment.
- Focus on keeping your balance and preventing your feet from touching each other.
- Walk the length of the path, then turn around and repeat.

Performing heel-to-toe walks regularly can help enhance balance, coordination, and joint stability, all essential for individuals with knee arthritis.

Quadriceps Stretch

Stretching the quadriceps muscles is vital for maintaining flexibility and reducing tension around the knee joint. The quadriceps are essential for knee extension and overall lower limb function.

Instructions:

- Stand with the soles of your feet approximately hip-width apart, if necessary, grip onto a solid surface for stability.
- Bring your heel near your buttocks while bending one knee.
- Reach back with your hand and grasp your ankle or shin, depending on your flexibility.
- Pull your heel softly to your buttocks to feel a stretch in the front of your thigh (quadriceps).
- Maintain the stretch for 20-30 seconds, being mindful not to arch your back.
- Release and switch to the other leg.

Performing the quadriceps stretch regularly can help maintain flexibility in the quadriceps muscles, reducing the risk of knee pain and improving overall knee function.

IT Band Stretch

A substantial band of connective tissue that extends along the circumference of the thigh is called the iliotibial (IT) band.

Stretching the IT band can help alleviate tightness and discomfort in the knee area.

Instructions:

- Stand with the soles of your feet approximately hip-width apart, with one foot placed slightly in front of the other.
- Cross the back leg behind the front leg, shifting your weight to the front leg.
- Lean your upper body to the opposite side of the back leg, feeling a stretch along the outer thigh and hip.
- Maintain the stretch for 20 to 30 seconds before switching to the opposite side.

Stretching the IT band regularly can help reduce tension and tightness in the outer thigh and knee area, promoting better knee arthritis management.

Conclusion: Balancing and flexibility exercises are essential components of a comprehensive knee arthritis management program.

Incorporating yoga and Tai Chi, single-leg stance and balance exercises, heel-to-toe walks, quadriceps stretch, and IT band stretches into your exercise routine can improve joint stability, enhance flexibility, and reduce the risk of falls.

These exercises are gentle on the knees, making them suitable for individuals with knee arthritis seeking to maintain joint health and overall mobility.

Remember to consult your healthcare professional before starting any new exercise program, especially if you have knee arthritis, to ensure that these exercises are safe and appropriate for your specific condition.

Regularly practicing balancing and flexibility exercises can enhance your knee arthritis management journey and experience the long-term benefits of improved joint function and overall well-being.

CHAPTER EIGHT: PAIN MANAGEMENT TECHNIQUES DURING EXERCISE

Experiencing knee pain during exercise can be discouraging and challenging for individuals with knee arthritis. However, with the proper pain management techniques, it is possible to continue exercising safely and effectively while minimizing discomfort.

This chapter will explore four essential pain management techniques for individuals with knee arthritis: applying heat and cold therapy, using assistive devices, modifying exercises for comfort, and incorporating breathing and relaxation techniques.

Applying Heat And Cold Therapy

Heat and cold therapy are simple yet effective methods for managing knee pain during and after exercise. Both treatments relieve inflammation, alleviate muscle tension, and soothe sore joints. Deciding when to use heat or cold therapy depends on the type of pain experienced.

Heat Therapy: Applying heat to the affected knee before exercise can help relax muscles and improve blood flow, preparing the joint for activity. Heat can also be beneficial after exercise to ease stiffness and promote muscle relaxation.

Instructions for Heat Therapy:

1. Use a thermal pad on the lowest setting or a warm, damp towel.
2. Apply the heat pack to the affected knee for 15-20 minutes.
3. Take breaks in between, and avoid falling asleep with the heat pack on to prevent burns.

Cold Therapy: Cold therapy reduces inflammation and numbs the area, making it an excellent option for post-exercise recovery when the knee may be swollen or tender.

Instructions for Cold Therapy:

1. Use a tiny cloth-wrapped bag of vegetables that are frozen or a cold pack.
2. For 15 to 20 minutes, place the injured knee on the cold pack.
3. Allow the knee to warm up to room temperature before reapplying the cold pack.

Remember, never apply heat or cold directly to the skin, and avoid using these therapies for too long to prevent skin damage. If you have circulatory issues or nerve damage, consult your healthcare professional before using heat or cold therapy.

Using Assistive Devices

Assistive devices can offer valuable support during exercise, easing knee strain and promoting proper alignment. These devices are especially beneficial for individuals with knee arthritis, as they can help reduce pain and prevent further damage to the joint.

Knee Braces: Knee braces provide stability and compression, helping to alleviate knee pain and reduce stress on the joint during exercise. There are different types of knee braces, including sleeves, hinged braces, and unloader braces, each designed to address specific knee issues.

Instructions for Using Knee Braces:

1. Consult your healthcare professional to determine the most suitable knee brace for your condition.
2. Follow the manufacturer's instructions on adequately wearing and adjusting the knee brace for optimal support.

3. Avoid wearing the knee brace too tightly, leading to discomfort and restricted blood flow.

Walking Aids: Mobility aids, such as canes or walking sticks, can assist individuals with knee arthritis maintain balance and stability during exercise. These aids can also help reduce the load on the affected knee, making walking and exercising less painful.

Instructions for Using Walking Aids:

1. Choose a walking aid that is the appropriate height for your comfort and needs.
2. Hold the walking aid on the opposite side of your affected knee to provide support and stability.
3. Practice using the walking aid before exercising to ensure you are comfortable and confident with its use.

Using assistive devices can significantly improve the exercise experience for individuals with knee arthritis, allowing them to engage in physical activities with reduced pain and improved joint support.

Modifying Exercises For Comfort

Modifying exercises is crucial to managing knee arthritis pain during physical activity. Making minor adjustments to the intensity, range of motion, and body position can help reduce knee stress while reaping the benefits of the exercise.

Low-Impact Exercises: Opt for low-impact exercises that are gentler on the joints, such as swimming, cycling, or using an elliptical machine. These activities provide an effective cardiovascular workout without subjecting the knees to excessive pressure.

Range of Motion: Avoid exercises that involve deep knee bends or sudden changes in direction, as these movements can exacerbate knee pain. Instead, focus on controlled and fluid motions that do not put undue stress on the joint.

Joint-Friendly Activities: Engage in activities that promote joint health, such as tai chi and yoga. These practices emphasize gentle movements, stretching, and strengthening without placing excessive strain on the knees.

Shorter Sessions: Consider breaking your exercise routine into shorter sessions throughout the day rather than engaging in prolonged, high-impact workouts. This approach can help manage knee arthritis pain and prevent overexertion.

Listen to Your Body: Pay attention to your body's signals and stop exercising if you experience significant pain or discomfort. As your knee arthritis treatment improves, it's critical to respect your restrictions and gradually elevate the intensity and length of your workouts.

Breathing And Relaxation Techniques

Incorporating breathing and relaxation techniques into your exercise routine can promote a sense of calm and reduce stress, contributing to better pain management during physical activity.

Deep Breathing: Practice deep breathing exercises before, during, and after exercise to promote relaxation and focus. Deep breathing can help lower tension in the body and calm the mind, making exercise more enjoyable and less stressful.

Instructions for Deep Breathing:

1. Find a comfortable seated or lying position.
2. Deeply inhale air into your lungs through your nose.
3. Release any tension or stress by inhaling through your mouth slowly and fully.
4. Repeat this deep breathing pattern for several minutes, allowing yourself to relax and center your thoughts.

Progressive Muscle Relaxation: Progressive muscle relaxation involves tensing and releasing different muscle groups to achieve peace and reduce muscle tension.

Instructions for Progressive Muscle Relaxation:

1. Look for a place that is calm and cozy to sit or to lie down.
2. Starting from your toes, tense the muscles in your feet and hold for a few seconds.
3. Let go of the tension and permit complete muscle relaxation.
4. Move on to the next muscle group, working your way up through your legs, abdomen, chest, arms, and face, repeating the tension and release pattern.

Mindfulness Meditations: Practicing mindfulness meditation can help you become more aware of your body and any sensations you may be experiencing during exercise. This awareness can aid in managing knee arthritis pain and preventing overexertion.

Instructions for Mindfulness Meditation:

1. Look for a place that is calm and cozy to sit or to lie down.

2. Pay attention to your breathing, impartially observing each inhalation and exhalation.

3. Redirect your attention back to your breath whenever your thoughts start to stray.

4. Expand your awareness to other sensations in your body, including any discomfort in the knees, acknowledging these sensations without trying to change them.

Incorporating breathing and relaxation techniques into your exercise routine can enhance your pain management strategies and promote a positive and calming exercise experience.

Conclusion: Pain management during exercise is essential for individuals with knee arthritis to continue engaging in physical activities safely and effectively. Heat and cold therapy can reduce inflammation and soothe sore joints, while assistive devices offer support and stability.

Modifying exercises for comfort and incorporating breathing and relaxation techniques can further enhance pain management and improve the exercise experience.

Remember that every individual's knee arthritis experience is unique, and it is crucial to consult with your healthcare professional before implementing any pain management techniques during exercise.

CHAPTER NINE: INCORPORATING LIFESTYLE CHANGES FOR ENHANCED RESULTS

In managing knee arthritis, exercise alone is not the sole answer. Embracing a holistic approach by incorporating lifestyle changes can significantly enhance the results and overall well-being. In this chapter, we will delve into four vital lifestyle changes that can complement exercises for knee arthritis: the role of diet, managing weight for joint health, improving sleep quality, and stress reduction strategies.

The Role of Diet In Knee Arthritis

A healthy diet that is balanced and rich in nutrients is essential for controlling knee arthritis. Certain foods possess anti-inflammatory properties and can help alleviate joint pain and inflammation.

On the other hand, some foods may exacerbate arthritis symptoms, leading to increased discomfort. Understanding the impact of diet on knee health can empower individuals to make informed choices for better arthritis management.

a. **Anti-Inflammatory Foods:** Incorporating anti-inflammatory foods into your diet can aid in reducing inflammation and managing knee arthritis pain. Antioxidants and other elements that assist joint health are abundant in these foods.

   Examples of Anti-Inflammatory Foods:

   - Salmon, mackerel, and sardines are examples of fatty fish that are rich in omega-3 as well as fatty acids.
   - Colorful fruits and vegetables, like berries, cherries, leafy greens, and broccoli, which are packed with antioxidants.
   - Nuts and seeds, including walnuts, almonds, and chia seeds, which provide healthy fats and plant-based protein.
   - Whole grains, such as brown rice, quinoa, and oats, are good sources of fiber and nutrients.

b. **Foods to Avoid or eat Less of:** Certain foods can trigger inflammation and worsen knee arthritis symptoms. Reducing the consumption of these foods can contribute to better arthritis management.

   Examples of Foods to Limit or Avoid:

- Processed and fried foods often contain trans fats and high levels of unhealthy fats.
- Sugary snacks and beverages, as excess sugar can lead to inflammation.
- White bread and pastries are examples of refined carbs that can quickly raise blood sugar levels.

c. **Hydration:** Staying adequately hydrated is essential for joint health. Water helps cushion and lubricate the joints, reducing friction and promoting smooth movement.

Instructions for Hydration:

- Throughout the day, take lots of water; aim for at least 8 to 10 cups.
- Limit the consumption of sugary and caffeinated beverages, as they can lead to dehydration.

Managing Weight For Joint Health

Maintaining a healthy weight is crucial for individuals with knee arthritis. Excess body weight stresses knee joints, leading to increased pain and discomfort. By managing weight through proper nutrition and regular exercise, individuals can significantly improve joint health and reduce the burden on their knees.

1. **Body Mass Index (BMI) and Ideal Weight:** Calculate your BMI to determine whether you are within a healthy weight range. Knowing your ideal weight can be a reference point for setting achievable weight management goals.

    Instructions for Calculating BMI:

    - Your height in square meters divided by your weight in kilos (BMI = weight [kg] / height [m]^2).
    - To establish if you are underweight, medium weight, overweight, or obese, correlate your measurements to the BMI categories.

2. **Balanced Caloric Intake:** Consuming a balanced number of calories is essential for weight management. Eating mindfully and avoiding overeating can contribute to maintaining a healthy weight.

    Instructions for Balanced Caloric Intake:

    - Be mindful of portion sizes, avoiding oversized servings.
    - Put an emphasis on nutrient-dense foods that offer vital vitamins and minerals without having a lot of calories.

3. **Regular Exercise:** Regular physical activity is not only beneficial for joint health but also for weight

management. As discussed in previous chapters, engaging in low-impact exercises can help burn calories without putting excessive strain on the knees.

Instructions for Regular Exercise:

- Plan to engage in moderate-intensity exercise for at least 150 minutes or 75 minutes of vigorous-intensity exercise.

- Find activities you enjoy to make exercise a sustainable and enjoyable part of your lifestyle.

Improving Sleep Quality

For general health and wellbeing, including joint health, quality sleep is essential. During sleep, the body undergoes essential repair processes, helping to reduce inflammation and restore energy levels. For individuals with knee arthritis, improving sleep quality can enhance the body's ability to manage pain and promote healing.

1. **Sleep Environment:** Creating a conducive sleep environment can significantly impact the quality of your sleep. Make sure your bedroom is peaceful, dark, and at a comfortable temperature for restful sleep.

   Instructions for Improving Sleep Environment:

- Invest in a comfortable mattress and supportive pillows that suit your sleep preferences.
- To filter out light that can keep you awake at night, use curtains that are blackout or an eye mask.
- Keep noise levels to a minimum, or consider using white noise machines to mask disruptive sounds.

2. **Establish a Sleep Routine:** Developing a consistent sleep routine can signal your body that it is time to wind down and prepare for rest. Better sleep patterns can be encouraged by waking up and going to bed at the same time each day.

Instructions for Establishing a Sleep Routine:
- Establish a relaxing nighttime ritual, such as reading a book, practicing relaxation exercises, or taking a warm bath.
- Avoid stimulating activities, such as electronic devices or intense exercise, close to bedtime.

3. **Manage Stress and Anxiety:** These can interfere with sleep quality. As discussed in the next section, incorporating stress reduction techniques can aid in improving sleep.

Instructions for Stress Management:

- Practice relaxation exercises before bedtime, such as deep breathing and mindfulness meditation.
- Think about keeping a diary to write down any worries or thoughts that may keep you awake.

Stress Reduction Strategies

Managing stress is essential for overall well-being, including arthritis management. Chronic stress can raise inflammation and make the symptoms of knee arthritis worse. Stress reduction strategies can positively impact joint health and overall quality of life.

1. **Mindfulness and Meditation:** Meditation and other mindfulness techniques can help people cultivate a calm disposition and lessen stress.

   Instructions for Mindfulness and Meditation:

- Find a place that is calm and relaxing for practicing mindfulness.

- Set aside a few minutes daily to focus on your breath and observe your thoughts without judgment.

2. **Physical Activity:** Regular physical activity, even low-impact exercises, can release endorphins, the body's natural mood elevators, and reduce stress.

Instructions for Physical Activity:

- Incorporate exercises from earlier chapters, such as gentle range of motion exercises and low-impact cardiovascular exercises, into your routine to reduce stress and boost mood.

3. **Social Support:** Connecting with friends, family, or support groups can provide emotional support and a sense of belonging, which can help alleviate stress.

   Instructions for Seeking Social Support:

- Make regular contact with loved ones by calling, using video chat, or meeting in person.

- Consider joining a local or online support group for individuals with knee arthritis to share experiences and coping strategies.

4. Time Management: Effectively managing time and setting realistic goals can reduce feelings of overwhelm and stress.

   Instructions for Time Management:

- Set tasks in order of importance and divide them into manageable steps to prevent feeling overwhelmed.

- Delegate tasks when possible to lighten the workload.

Conclusion: Incorporating lifestyle changes into your knee arthritis management can enhance results and improve overall well-being. The role of diet in reducing inflammation, managing weight for joint health, improving sleep quality, and implementing stress reduction strategies are all essential aspects of holistic arthritis management.

By combining these lifestyle changes with the exercises and pain management techniques discussed in previous chapters, individuals can take charge of their knee arthritis journey and experience the benefits of a comprehensive and balanced approach to joint health.

CHAPTER TEN: OVERCOMING CHALLENGES AND STAYING MOTIVATED

In managing knee arthritis through exercises and lifestyle changes, it is essential to acknowledge that challenges and setbacks are natural parts of the process. Overcoming these obstacles and staying motivated is crucial for long-term success and improved joint health.

This chapter will explore four vital strategies to navigate challenges and maintain motivation: dealing with flare-ups and setbacks, building a supportive network, tracking progress and celebrating success, and setting long-term goals for sustainable results.

Dealing With Flare-ups And Setbacks

Dealing with flare-ups and setbacks is an inevitable part of managing knee arthritis. Flare-ups occur when arthritis symptoms, such as pain and inflammation, suddenly worsen. On the other hand, setbacks may arise from overexertion, increased stress, or neglecting proper self-care. It is crucial to approach these challenges positively and adopt coping strategies.

1. **Listen to Your Body:** Pay close attention to your body and recognize the signs of a flare-up or setback. If you experience increased pain, stiffness, or swelling in your knees, it may indicate that you need to modify your exercise routine or take a break.

2. **Rest and Recovery:** When faced with a flare-up or setback, prioritize rest and allow your body time to recover. Resting your knees and avoiding high-impact activities can help reduce inflammation and prevent further aggravation of symptoms.

3. **Modify Your Exercise Routine:** Adjusting your exercise routine during a flare-up or setback is essential. Focus on low-impact exercises, gentle range of motion exercises, and flexibility routines to maintain joint mobility without exacerbating symptoms.

4. **Consult Your Healthcare Professional:** If you experience persistent or severe flare-ups or setbacks, consult your healthcare professional for guidance. They can assess your condition and recommend appropriate adjustments to your arthritis management plan.

5. **Maintain a Positive Mindset:** Feeling discouraged during flare-ups and setbacks is normal, but maintaining

a positive mindset can help you overcome these challenges. Remember your progress so far, and stay committed to your overall health and well-being.

Building A Supportive Network

A supportive network can significantly impact your motivation and ability to manage knee arthritis effectively. Surrounding yourself with individuals who understand your challenges and provide encouragement can boost your confidence and keep you on track with your exercise and lifestyle goals.

- **Seek Support from Family and Friends:** Share your arthritis journey with your close family and friends. Their understanding and encouragement can provide the emotional support you need to stay motivated.

- **Join a Support Group:** Consider joining a local or online support group specifically for individuals with knee arthritis. Engaging with others who share similar experiences can be empowering and offer valuable insights and coping strategies.

- **Work with a Physical Therapist:** Enlist the help of a physical therapist who specializes in arthritis management. They can create a personalized exercise program, guide you through proper form and technique, and provide ongoing support.

- **Communicate with Your Healthcare Team:** Keep your healthcare team informed about your progress, challenges, and goals. Regular communication ensures that your treatment plan remains tailored to your needs.

- **Celebrate Your Achievements Together:** Celebrate your milestones and achievements with your support network. Whether completing a new exercise routine or improving joint mobility, recognizing your progress can reinforce your motivation.

Tracking Progress And Celebrating Success

Tracking your progress and celebrating your success is a powerful way to stay motivated on your knee arthritis management journey. Setting tangible goals and acknowledging your achievements can provide a sense of accomplishment and drive you to continue working towards improved joint health.

- **Set Realistic and Specific Goals:** Establish clear and achievable goals for your arthritis management, such as increasing the number of minutes spent exercising each week or reducing the frequency of knee pain.

- **Keep a Journal:** Maintain a journal to track your exercise routines, diet, and any changes in your arthritis symptoms. This journal can be a valuable resource for identifying patterns and progress over time.

- **Use Fitness Apps and Devices:** Utilize fitness apps or wearable devices to monitor your exercise activity, heart rate, and overall progress. These tools can offer real-time feedback and provide added motivation.

- **Embrace Non-Scale Victories:** Recognize and celebrate non-scale victories, such as improved flexibility, reduced pain during specific movements, or increased energy levels. These achievements are just as significant as reaching a numerical goal.

- **Reward Yourself:** Create a system of rewards for reaching your objectives. When you reach a milestone, treat yourself to something enjoyable, such as a favorite activity or a relaxing spa day.

Setting Long-term Goals For Sustainable Results

To maintain motivation and sustain positive results, it is crucial to set long-term goals that encompass your arthritis management journey. Long-term goals provide direction and purpose, helping you stay focused and committed to making lasting lifestyle changes.

1. **Create a Vision Board:** Develop a vision board representing your long-term health and well-being goals. Include images and words that inspire you and remind you of the positive outcomes you are working towards.

2. **Break Goals into Smaller Steps:** Long-term goals can feel overwhelming, but breaking them down into smaller, manageable steps can make them more achievable. Focus on accomplishing one step at a time, and celebrate each milestone.

3. **Adapt and Adjust:** Be flexible with your goals and be willing to adapt them as needed. Life circumstances may change, and your arthritis management plan may require adjustments to remain effective.

4. **Focus on Sustainable Habits:** Prioritize sustainable habits you can maintain over time. Rather than pursuing quick fixes, build lasting lifestyle changes supporting your knee arthritis management.

5. **Keep Learning and Growing:** Stay informed about the latest research and developments in arthritis management. Continuously educate yourself about exercise techniques, nutrition, and self-care practices that can enhance your overall well-being.

Conclusion: Overcoming challenges and staying motivated are integral parts of managing knee arthritis through exercises and lifestyle changes. Dealing with flare-ups and setbacks requires listening to your body, practicing self-compassion, and seeking support. Building a supportive network of family, friends, healthcare professionals, and support groups can empower you to face challenges head-on.

Tracking progress, celebrating successes, and setting long-term goals are powerful tools for maintaining motivation and sustaining positive results. By adopting a comprehensive and proactive strategy for managing knee arthritis, you can achieve improved joint health, enhanced quality of life, and a future filled with vitality and well-being.

CONCLUSION

In the pages of this book, we have explored a comprehensive guide to managing knee arthritis through exercises and lifestyle changes. Throughout this journey, we have delved into the understanding of knee arthritis, its types, causes, and symptoms. We have learned how to diagnose knee arthritis accurately to embark on a targeted and effective management plan.

From a gentle range of motion exercises to low-impact cardiovascular exercises, we have discovered a plethora of exercises that can promote joint health, flexibility, and overall well-being.

Yet, this book goes beyond mere exercises; it embraces a holistic approach to knee arthritis management. We have explored the significance of diet, weight management, sleep quality, and stress reduction, understanding that these lifestyle changes complement exercises to deliver enhanced results.

By nourishing our bodies with anti-inflammatory foods, maintaining a healthy weight, and engaging in mindful practices, we have empowered ourselves to take charge of our joint health and foster sustainable progress.

We have encountered challenges and setbacks in our journey, acknowledging them as natural parts of the process. Armed with resilience and determination, we have learned to navigate these obstacles gracefully. Through rest, modification, and the support of our network, we have triumphed over adversity and remained steadfast on our path to better joint health.

The power of a supportive network cannot be underestimated. Family, friends, healthcare professionals, and support groups have rallied around us, providing encouragement, empathy, and valuable guidance. We have shared our victories, celebrated our achievements, and found solace in a community that understands our struggles.

We have learned the importance of tracking progress, setting realistic goals, and celebrating milestones. From small triumphs to non-scale victories, we have recognized the significance of every step taken in the right direction. We have discovered that sustainable habits and adaptability are the foundations of lasting progress, continuously learning and growing on our journey to improved joint health.

As we reach the end of this book, let us embrace the wisdom and knowledge we have gained. May we embark on our knee arthritis management journey with newfound determination, armed with exercises and lifestyle changes to pave the way for a brighter, healthier future. Together, let us stride confidently towards a life filled with vitality, well-being, and the freedom to move quickly.

Remember, the journey does not end here; it has just begun. Let this book be a steadfast companion, guiding us on our path to better knee health and inspiring us to live life to the fullest. Empowered by knowledge, supported by community, and motivated by our determination, we can overcome any obstacle that comes our way.

With unwavering hope and a commitment to a healthier tomorrow, let us take the lessons from these pages and create a life of strength, joy, and resilience. As we embrace each day with gratitude and optimism, let us be the architects of our knee arthritis management, carving out a future of boundless possibilities.

May this book serve as a beacon of hope and guidance for all those seeking relief and empowerment in the face of knee arthritis. Together, we can conquer the challenges, celebrate the victories, and rewrite the narrative of knee arthritis, forging a path to a life of comfort, vitality, and happiness.

Printed in Great Britain
by Amazon

46317346R00056